"We are as trees.
To be found in all shapes
and sizes.

Some can be apple, some
maybe pear.

Sometimes you blossom
and sometimes you may fall.

Although different, we are
all beautiful"

With the right wind behind
you, to help you stand tall,
your beauty and grace will
conquer all.

Angie Bowers

Page 8....90 Day Countdown & Mood
Tracker....If you are a happy tree, then
fill in your day face with a smile....
Or not! More Smiles are a good sign
you're on track and in balance with
your weight loss.

Authors: Jonathan & Angela Bowers
Cover Photograph: Shutterstock

HOW TO SET UP YOUR FOOD DIARY PAGE

This 3 Month Food Diary has been designed so it is compatible with any **Diet Plan** or **Formula** Simply use the blank columns on each page to match your plan. For example: If you are tracking your Protein, Fibre, Carbs and Fats you would set up your page to look like this ….

Protein	Carbs	Fibre	Fats	

And if you are following a "Club Diet" like Slimming World (TM) or Weight Watchers (TM) for example, your blank headers would be filled in with the groups food key words like "Free Food" or "Red or Green" and so on.

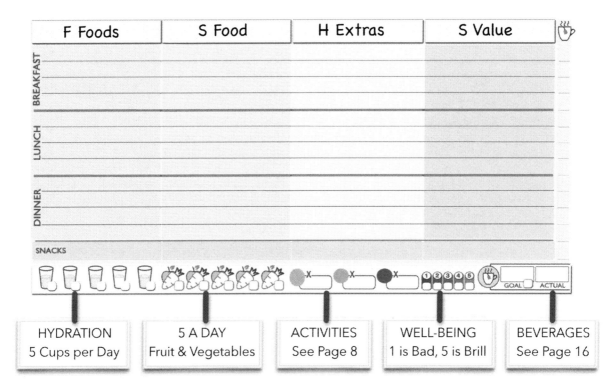

| | HYDRATION 5 Cups per Day | 5 A DAY Fruit & Vegetables | ACTIVITIES See Page 8 | WELL-BEING 1 is Bad, 5 is Brill | BEVERAGES See Page 16 |

Authors: Jonathan & Angela Bowers
Cover Photograph: Shutterstock

CONTENTS

ACTIVITY

Remember, tracking your activity and exercise is just as important as tracking your food. Exercise is a great way to burn calories and speed up weight loss, so we have built in an activity and exercise tracker - Please read page 8, so each day you can log your activities.

You will be able to look back and see how far you have come!

WELCOME TO YOUR NEW DIARY

Hello and welcome to your New Food Diary. This Diary is compatible with any food plan, and you will soon find it a super aid in your quest to lose weight. We are positive that using this Diary will become part of your day, and the helpful pages will help you keep on track, focused and in control.

If you have any questions please don't hesitate to get in touch via our website or our Facebook page.

www.thecalorieclub.com
www.facebook.com/thecalorieclub

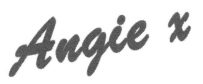

Please see pages 63 & 64 for information about our amazing exercise plan.
It's a real exercise plan for real people! www.thebodyplanplus.com

ABOUT ME

ME

Write down the things I like. What makes me, me?

_____

_____

_____

_____

_____

WHY

Write down why I want to make changes in my life.

_____

_____

_____

_____

_____

GOALS

What are my goals... What motivates me?

_____

_____

_____

_____

PLAN

Have something to look forward to... My plan are:

RELAX

What am I going to do to relax and unwind?

HELP!

Who can I talk to, and who is going to help me?

"We are as trees.
To be found in all
shapes and sizes.
Although different,
we are all beautiful"

MEASUREMENT TRACKER

When measuring yourself with the measuring tape, the tape should fit snugly against the surface of your skin. It should not press into the skin at any point. When wrapped around you, the measuring tape should be parallel with the floor, and not askew. When measuring your bust/chest, you'll get the best results if both arms are at your side. You may need assistance for this!

When doing your measurements, measure at the same point each time. Getting the same result, does not mean you haven't lost any weight. Remember your measurements are only guide lines. Measure yourself every other week.

	Neck	Bust	Waist	Hips	Arm Top (R)	Arm Top (L)	Thighs (R)	Thighs (L)	Calf (R)	Calf (L)
W 1										
W 2										
W 4										
W 6										
W 8										
W 10										
W 12										
W 13										

WEIGHT TRACKER & GRAPH

The best time of the day to weigh and measure yourself, is first thing in the morning after you have been to the toilet. Place your scales on an even surface, remove any clothing. Enter Week 1 into the box on your graph.

WEEK 2 RESULT		WEEK 3 RESULT		WEEK 4 RESULT		WEEK 5 RESULT		WEEK 6 RESULT		WEEK 7 RESULT	
Weigh in	18st 11 lbs	Weigh in	18st 3½ lbs	Weigh in	17st 13½ lbs	Weigh in	17st 10 lbs	Weigh in		Weigh in	
		Loss	7½ lbs	Loss	4 lbs	Loss	3½ lbs	Loss		Loss	

WEEK 8 RESULT		WEEK 9 RESULT		WEEK 10 RESULT		WEEK 11 RESULT		WEEK 12 RESULT		WEEK 13 RESULT	
Weigh in		Weigh in		Weigh in		Weigh in		Weigh in		Weigh in	
Loss		Loss		Loss		Loss		Loss		Loss	

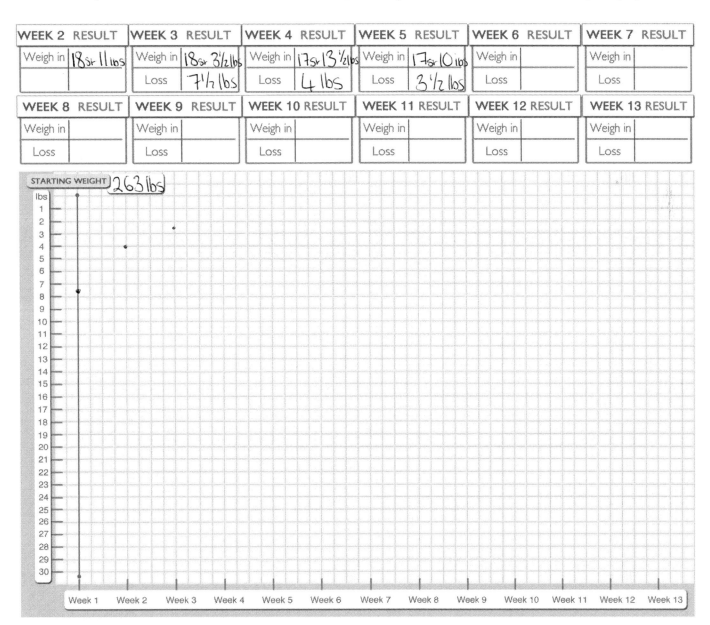

STARTING WEIGHT 263 lbs

NOTES & DOODLES

----

90 DAY COUNTDOWN & MOOD TRACKER

TO DO'S & REMINDERS

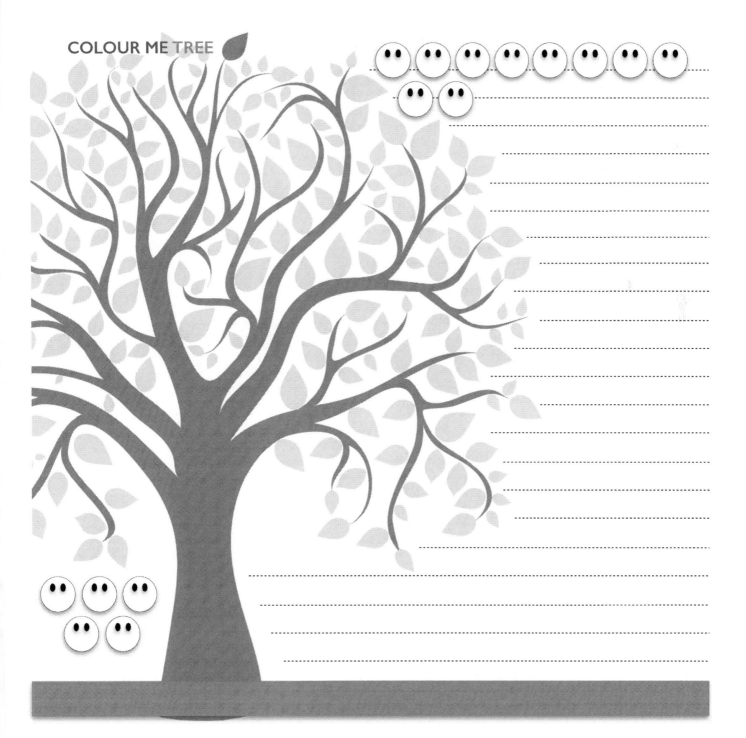

COLOUR ME TREE

ACTIVITIES & EXERCISE

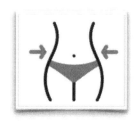

It is better to burn off calories than starve them off… So lets get active!

At the bottom of your Food Diary Pages you will see your activity icons.

GREEN is Light Activities / Exercise
PINK is Moderate Activities / Exercise
RED is Intensive Activities / Exercise

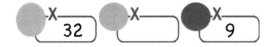

Make a note of the number of times you have been active throughout the day, in minutes.
For example: If you do 32 minutes light activities, you would put (32) next to the *GREEN* circle. And likewise, if you perform 9 minute Intense Activities/Exercise you would put a (9) next to the *RED* circle.

The Higher the number for each day the better!
Take this information and copy it onto your "Activity Page" opposite. This is a quick reference guide for you to see the increases in your activity and duration. Over the forthcoming weeks you should see the numbers get higher and higher.

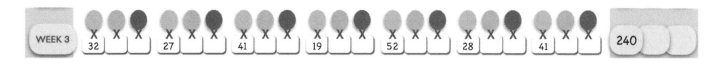

Example Light Activities: 32 + 27 + 41 + 19 + 52 + 28 + 41 = 240

You should also start to see more numbers appearing next to the RED circle (intense) Your daily total number should also start to get increases, even it's it more LIGHT activities performed. **IT ALL ADDS UP!**

Activities like walking and housework would be considered "Light Activities" (Green)
Exercises like Jumping Jacks and Mountain Climbs would be considered "Intensive Exercises" (Red)
For an amazing exercise plan, please see inside back cover.

QUICK REFERENCE ACTIVITY AND EXERCISE RECORD

	MONDAY	TUESDAY	WEDNESDAY	THURSDAY	FRIDAY	SATURDAY	SUNDAY	GRAND TOTALS
WEEK 1								
WEEK 2								
WEEK 3								
WEEK 4								
WEEK 5								
WEEK 6								
WEEK 7								
WEEK 8								
WEEK 9								
WEEK 10								
WEEK 11								
WEEK 12								
WEEK 13								

SHOPPING LIST MUST HAVES

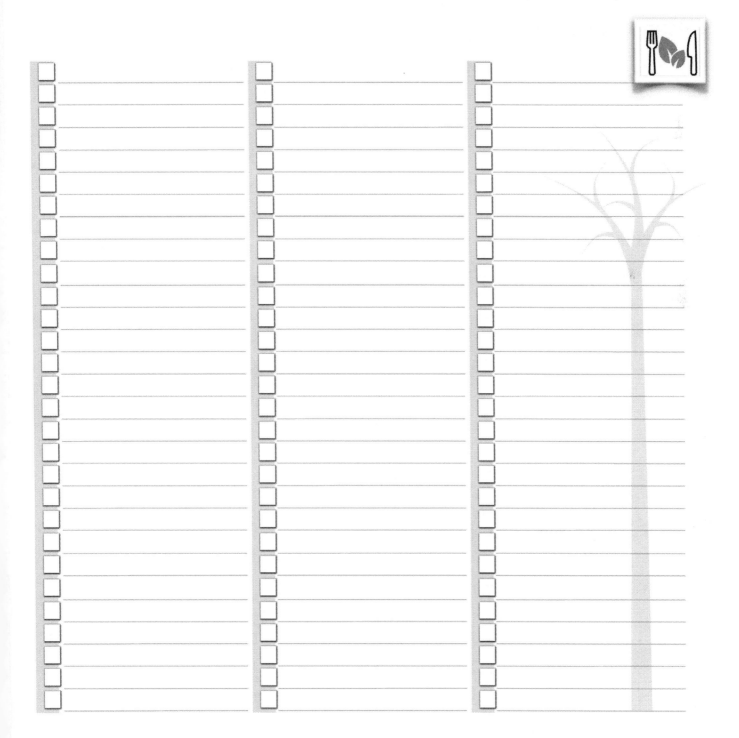

MONDAY | BREAKFAST | LUNCH | DINNER

TUESDAY | BREAKFAST | LUNCH | DINNER

WEDNESDAY | BREAKFAST | LUNCH | DINNER

THURSDAY | BREAKFAST | LUNCH | DINNER

FRIDAY | BREAKFAST | LUNCH | DINNER

SATURDAY | BREAKFAST | LUNCH | DINNER

SUNDAY | BREAKFAST | LUNCH | DINNER

MEAL PLANNER WEEKS

BREAKFAST	LUNCH	DINNER	MONDAY

BREAKFAST	LUNCH	DINNER	TUESDAY

BREAKFAST	LUNCH	DINNER	WEDNESDAY

BREAKFAST	LUNCH	DINNER	THURSDAY

BREAKFAST	LUNCH	DINNER	FRIDAY

BREAKFAST	LUNCH	DINNER	SATURDAY

BREAKFAST	LUNCH	DINNER	SUNDAY

MONDAY	BREAKFAST	LUNCH	DINNER

TUESDAY	BREAKFAST	LUNCH	DINNER

WEDNESDAY	BREAKFAST	LUNCH	DINNER

THURSDAY	BREAKFAST	LUNCH	DINNER

FRIDAY	BREAKFAST	LUNCH	DINNER

SATURDAY	BREAKFAST	LUNCH	DINNER

SUNDAY	BREAKFAST	LUNCH	DINNER

MEAL PLANNER WEEKS

BREAKFAST	LUNCH	DINNER	MONDAY

BREAKFAST	LUNCH	DINNER	TUESDAY

BREAKFAST	LUNCH	DINNER	WEDNESDAY

BREAKFAST	LUNCH	DINNER	THURSDAY

BREAKFAST	LUNCH	DINNER	FRIDAY

BREAKFAST	LUNCH	DINNER	SATURDAY

BREAKFAST	LUNCH	DINNER	SUNDAY

TICKS & BEVERAGES

Your beverages are just as important as your meals. Lots of people forget that beverages contain calories, or simply say "They don't count", however, they do!

Some people drink more beverages than others. This may be a work environment factor or simply drinking becomes more of a habit rather than a need.

If we all took in fluids for our needs only, we would only drink water. This would be a good thing, but we don't drink to simply nourish and hydrate our bodies anymore, we drink for flavour, enjoyment and to socialise.

Beverages taste nice and supply us with that little boost or kick we're looking for. The most common hot beverages are, you guessed it, tea, coffee and hot chocolate. For the younger generation it has to be fizzy drinks or an "Iced Frape - something".

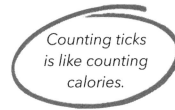

Counting ticks is like counting calories.

27 Calories
+
27 Calories
+
27 Calories

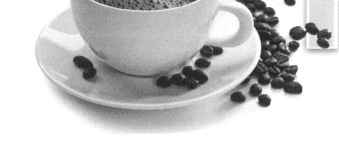

The reason I ask you to place a tick on your diary page each time you have a beverage is so you can see at a glance how many you're having during a single day. ***Morning, Afternoon & Evening.***

You may be shocked at the amount you're having, and reducing your beverages alone may be all the difference you're looking for to lose weight - Or it will at least go a long way to help!

Simply looking at the number of ticks on your page may give you a true picture to whether you are just having to many, or too many in one particular part of the day.

You may be able to say to yourself - *No more coffees in the morning*, or I will reduce this by half!

REDUCING YOUR BEVERAGES OVER TIME

I suggest for the first week of your diet you stick with you normal number of beverages. Then look back at the end of the week and find the pattern to see how you can realistically reduce the number. You don't want to lose too much of something you love, so start by setting a lower goal target and work it from there.

You will be amazed at how reducing your beverages has a marked impact on your weight loss, especially if you have sugar in your tea or coffee.

If you do have sugar in your tea or coffee and you are counting calories, use a measuring spoon instead of a teaspoon. A tea spoon of sugar can vary so much that over time your calorie count can be out by a lot!

Your spoonful may be bigger than mine!

A spoonful of sugar (1tsp 4.2g) is 16 calories. But is your spoonful 16 calories or more? There could be a 5 to 15 calorie difference if your spoonful is heaped. Times this by ten cups and your calorie count is out by as much as 150 calories! (1050 calories per week).

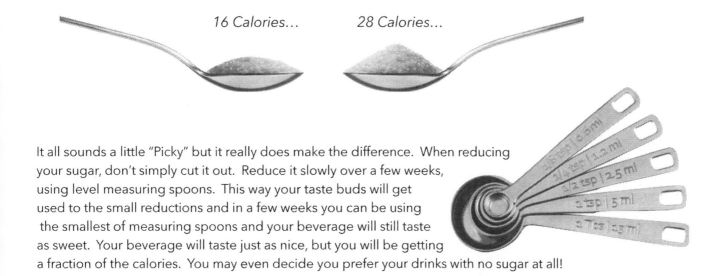

16 Calories...   *28 Calories...*

It all sounds a little "Picky" but it really does make the difference. When reducing your sugar, don't simply cut it out. Reduce it slowly over a few weeks, using level measuring spoons. This way your taste buds will get used to the small reductions and in a few weeks you can be using the smallest of measuring spoons and your beverage will still taste as sweet. Your beverage will taste just as nice, but you will be getting a fraction of the calories. You may even decide you prefer your drinks with no sugar at all!

Speed	free	HE	SYNS
BREAKFAST		A	
		A	
		B	
LUNCH			
DINNER			
SNACKS			

Glasses of water: ☐ ☐ ☐ ☐ ☐ Vegetables: 🥕 🥕 🥕 🥕 🥕 ●X ☐ ●X ☐ ●X ☐ 1 2 3 4 5 GOAL ☐ ACTUAL ☐

BREAKFAST			
LUNCH			
DINNER			
SNACKS			

Glasses of water: ☐ ☐ ☐ ☐ ☐ Vegetables: 🥕 🥕 🥕 🥕 🥕 ●X ☐ ●X ☐ ●X ☐ 1 2 3 4 5 GOAL ☐ ACTUAL ☐

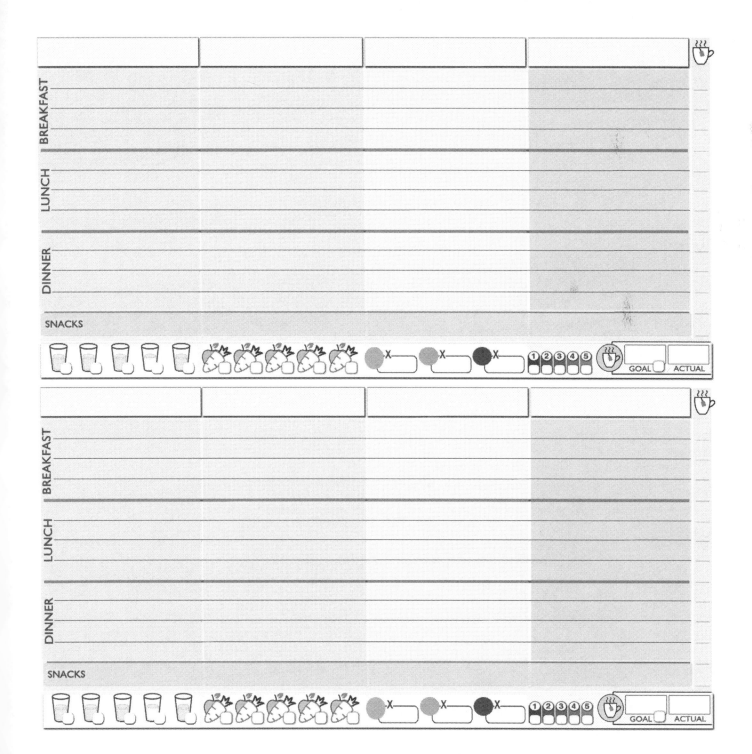

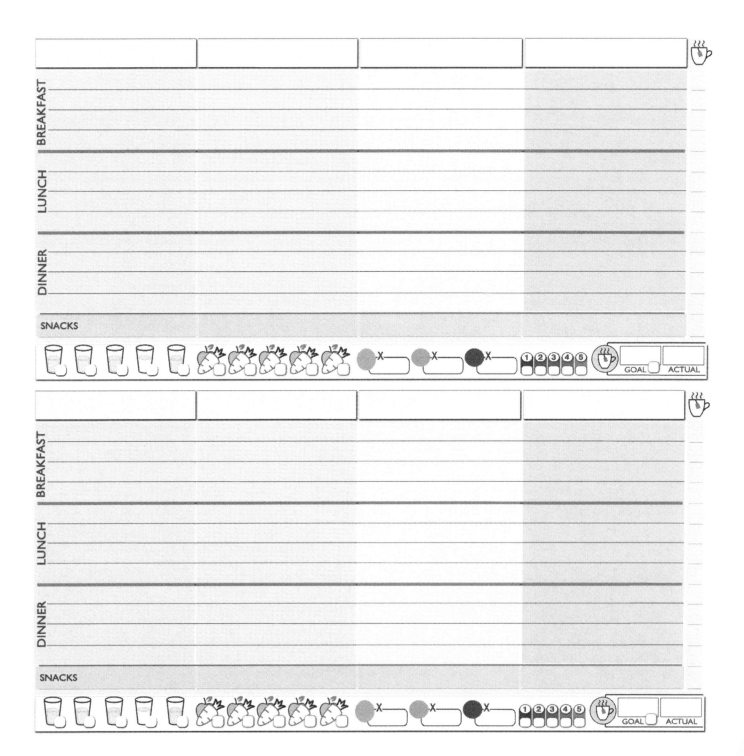

BREAKFAST

LUNCH

DINNER

SNACKS

GOAL ACTUAL

BREAKFAST

LUNCH

DINNER

SNACKS

GOAL ACTUAL

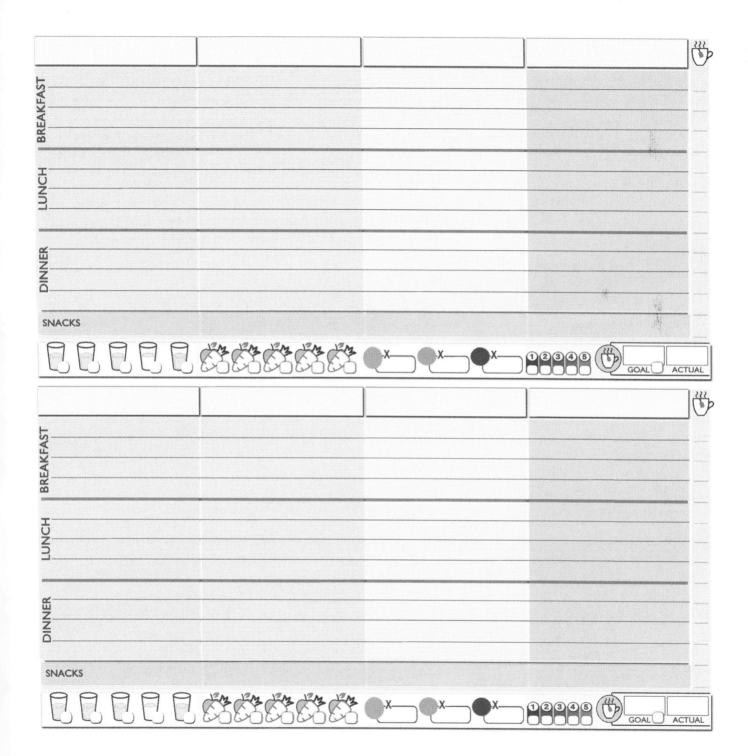

BREAKFAST

LUNCH

DINNER

SNACKS

GOAL   ACTUAL

BREAKFAST

LUNCH

DINNER

SNACKS

GOAL   ACTUAL

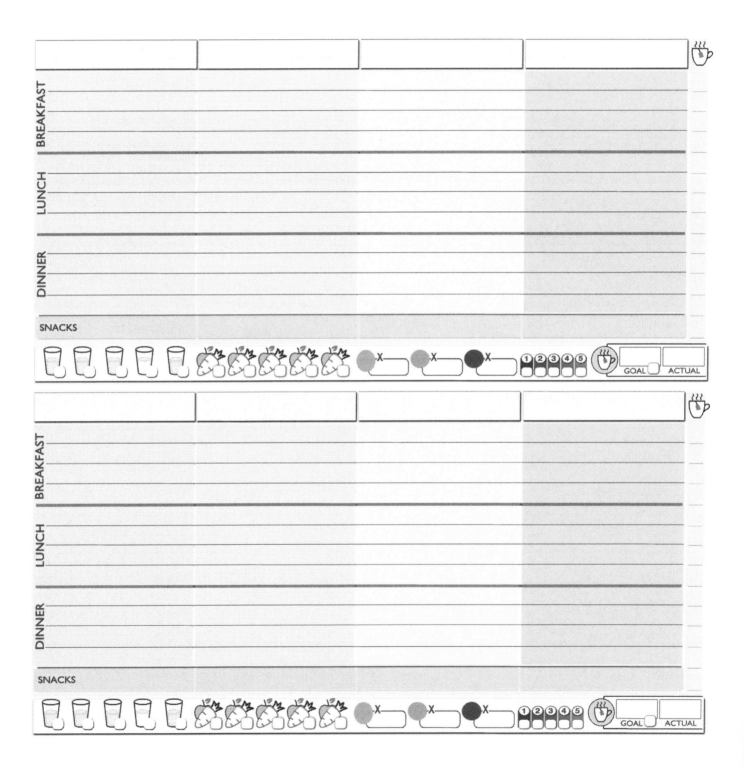

BREAKFAST

LUNCH

DINNER

SNACKS

GOAL   ACTUAL

BREAKFAST

LUNCH

DINNER

SNACKS

GOAL   ACTUAL

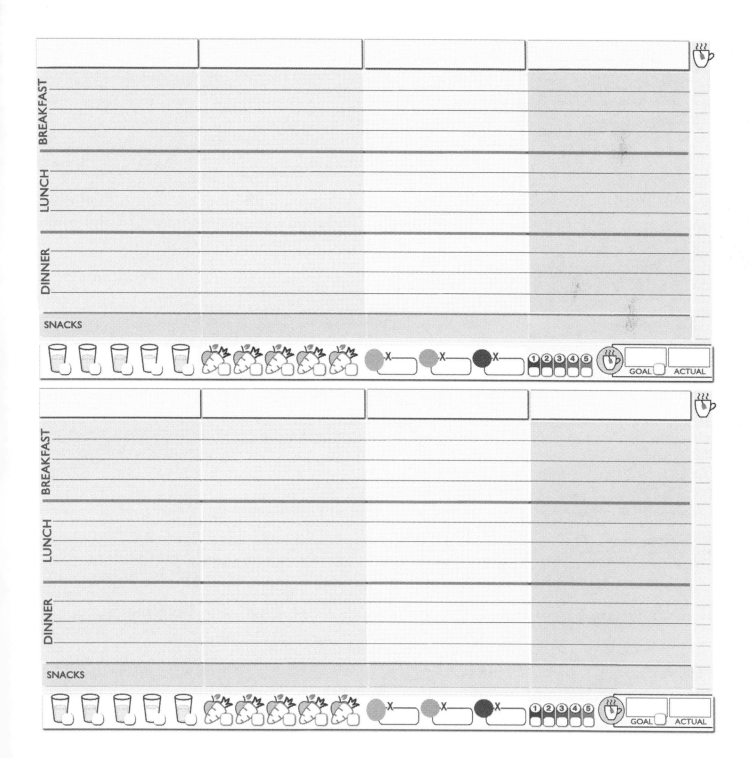

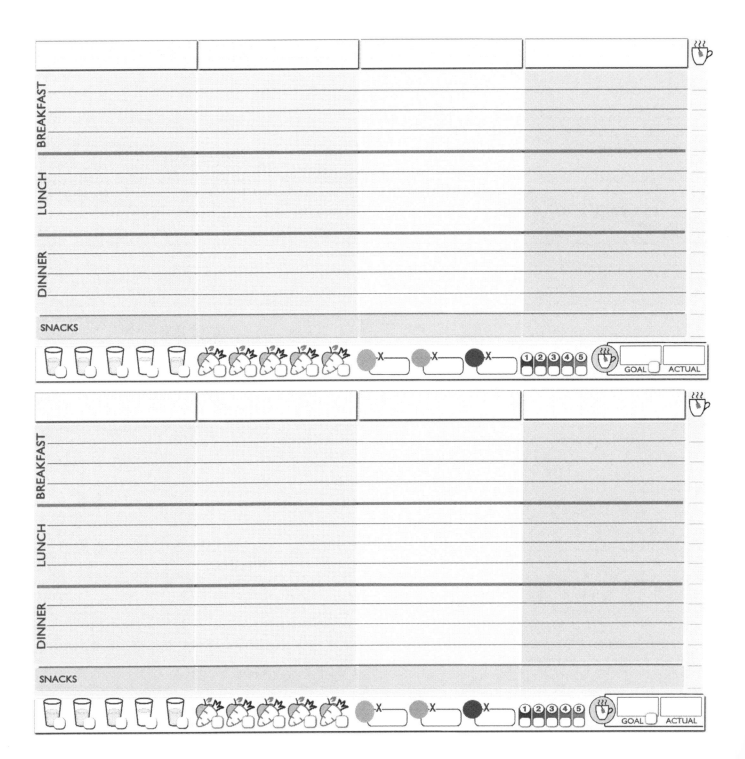

BREAKFAST

LUNCH

DINNER

SNACKS

GOAL   ACTUAL

BREAKFAST

LUNCH

DINNER

SNACKS

GOAL   ACTUAL

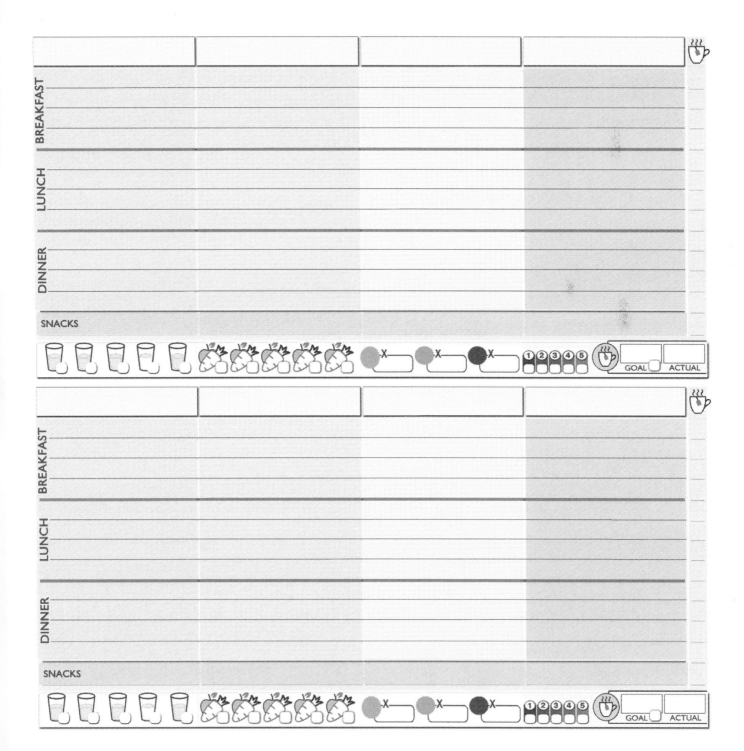

BREAKFAST

LUNCH

DINNER

SNACKS

GOAL   ACTUAL

BREAKFAST

LUNCH

DINNER

SNACKS

GOAL   ACTUAL

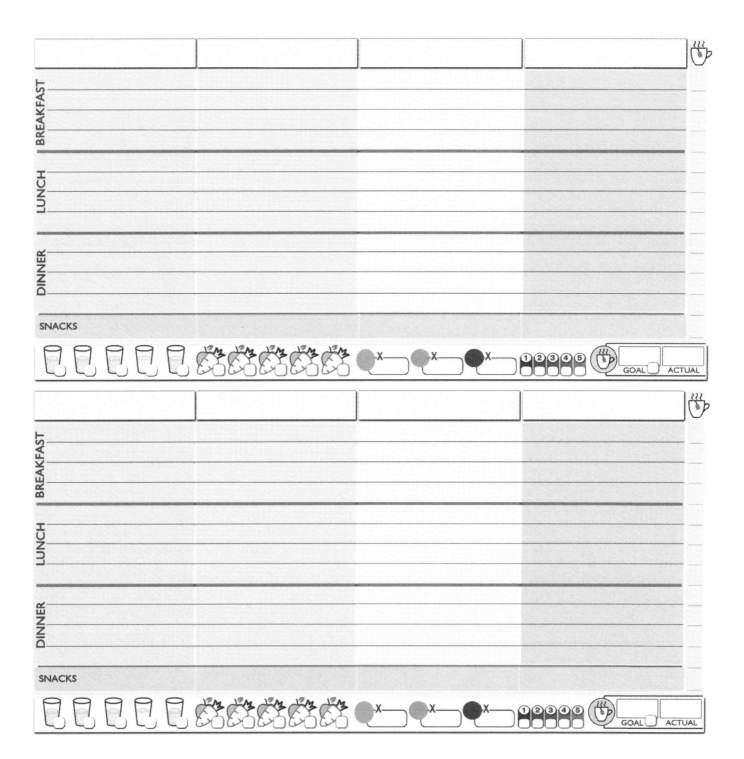

BREAKFAST

LUNCH

DINNER

SNACKS

GOAL   ACTUAL

BREAKFAST

LUNCH

DINNER

SNACKS

GOAL   ACTUAL

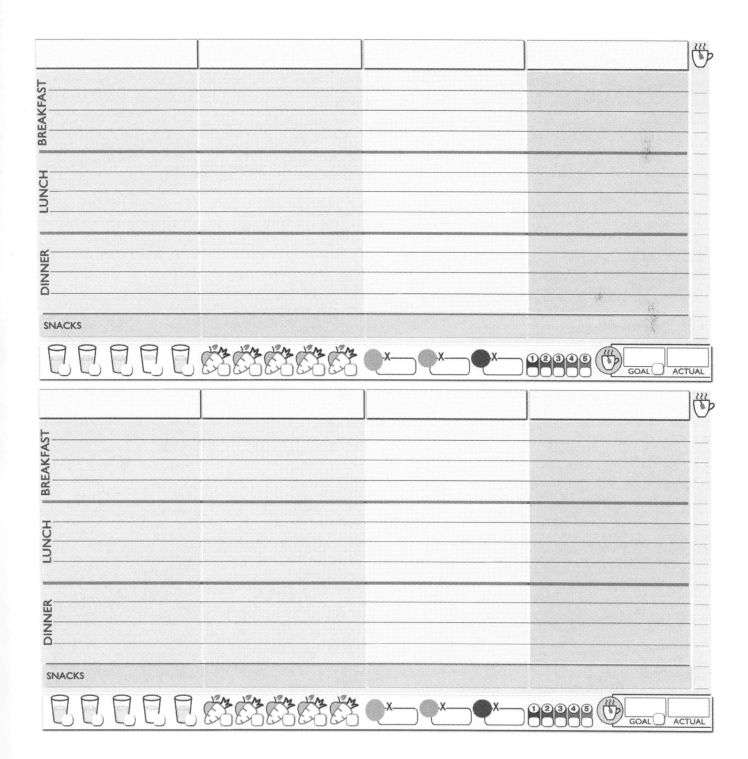

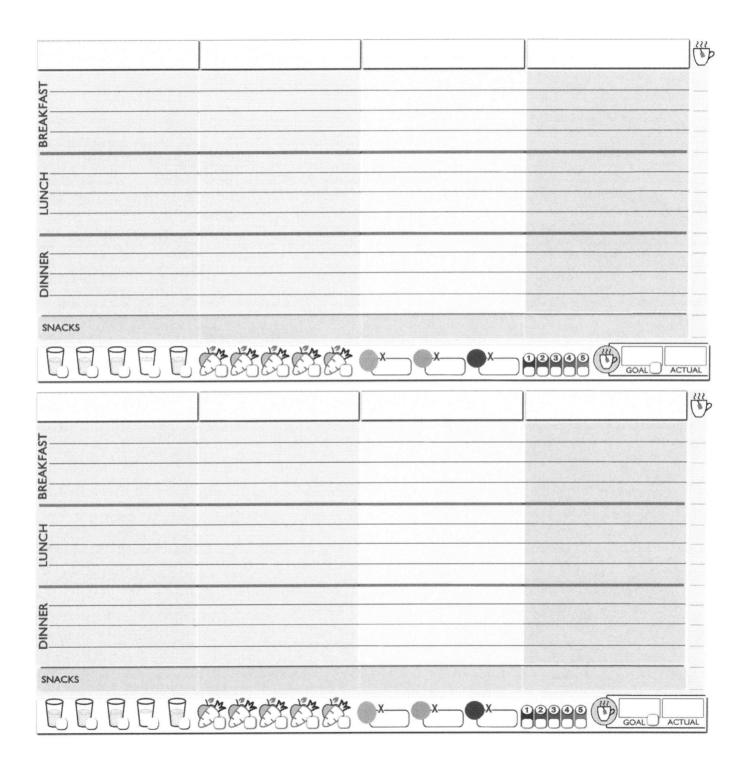

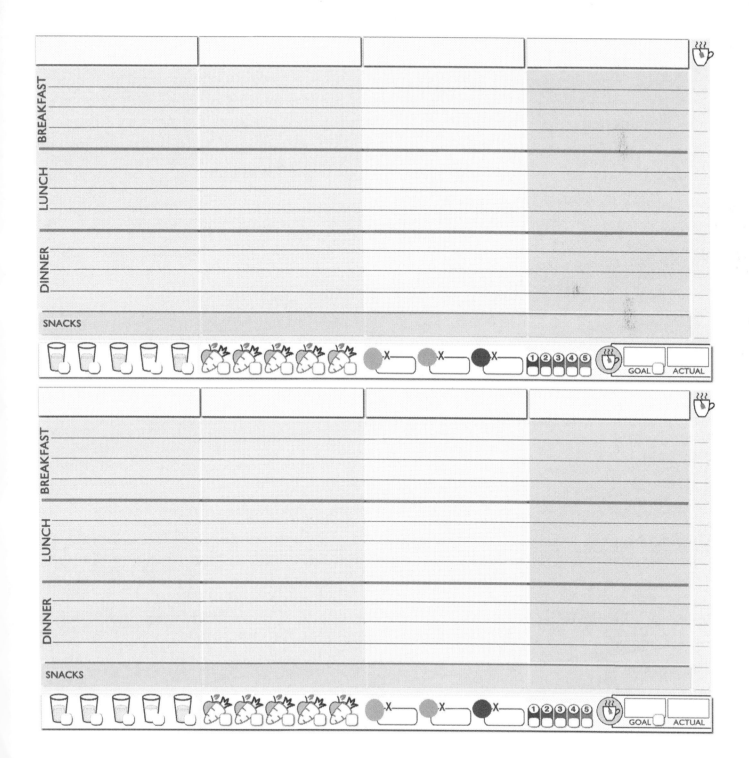

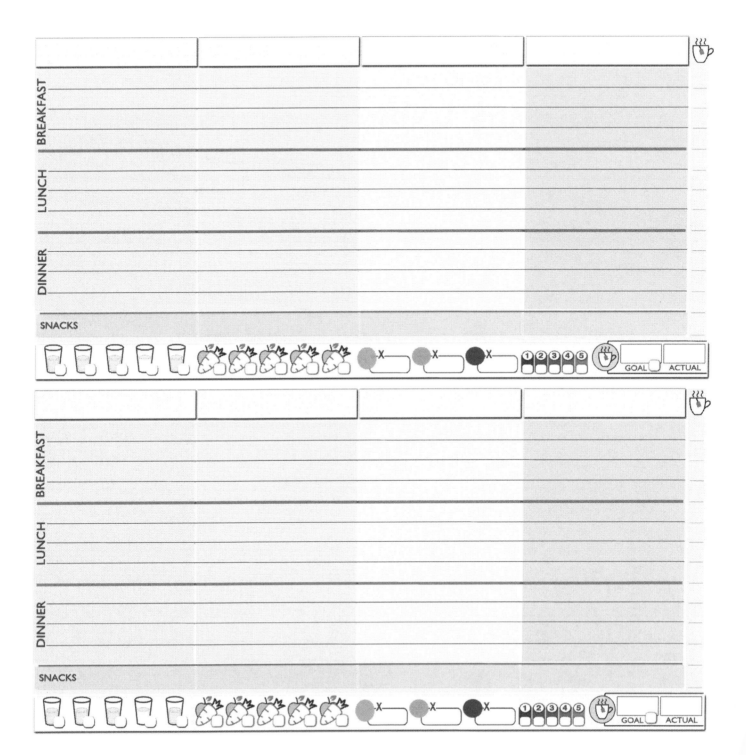

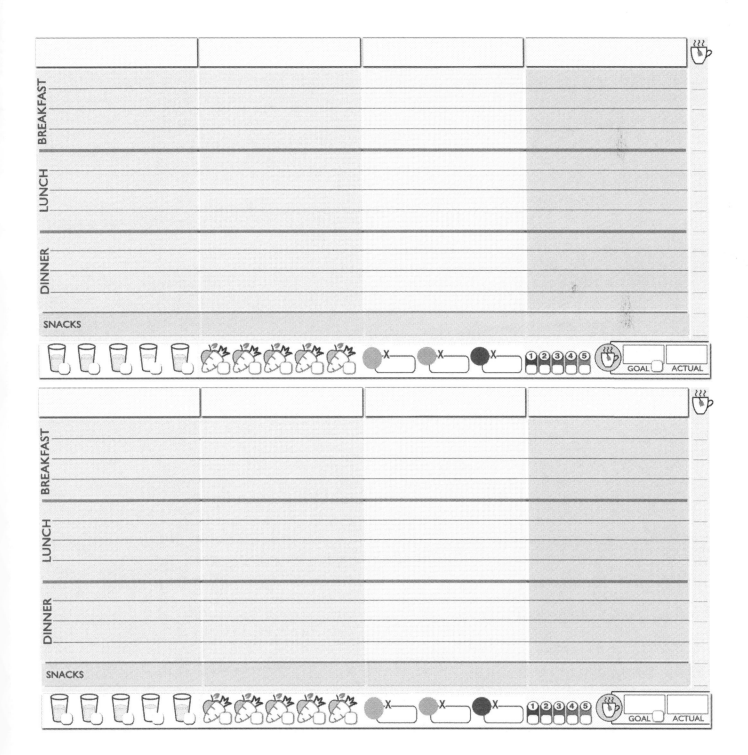

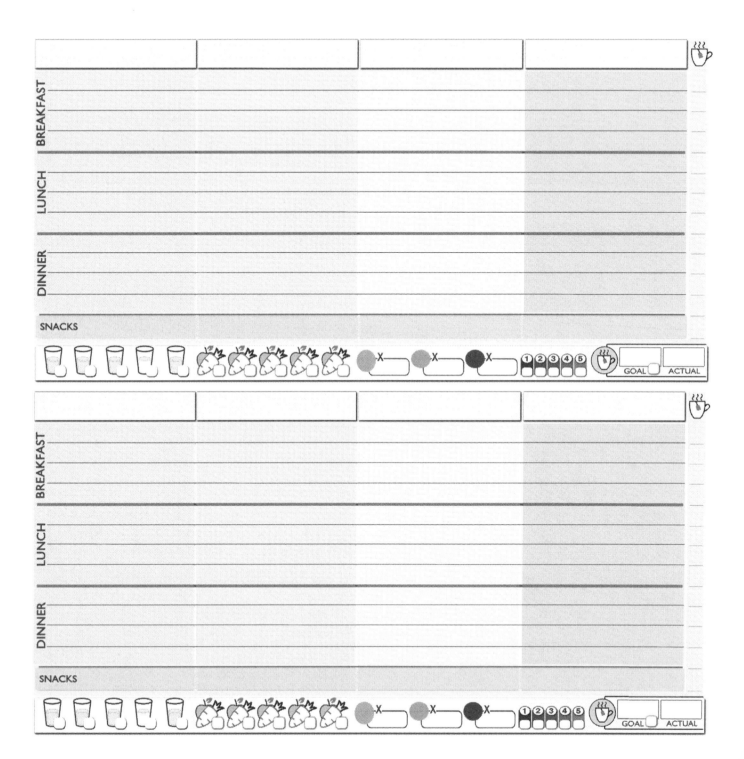

BREAKFAST

LUNCH

DINNER

SNACKS

GOAL   ACTUAL

BREAKFAST

LUNCH

DINNER

SNACKS

GOAL   ACTUAL

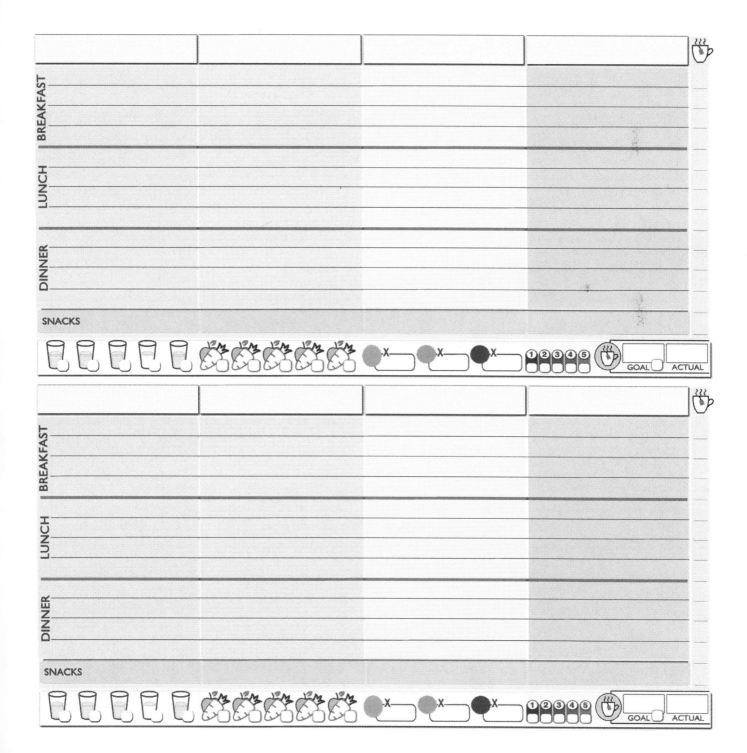

BREAKFAST

LUNCH

DINNER

SNACKS

GOAL   ACTUAL

1 2 3 4 5

BREAKFAST

LUNCH

DINNER

SNACKS

1 2 3 4 5

GOAL   ACTUAL

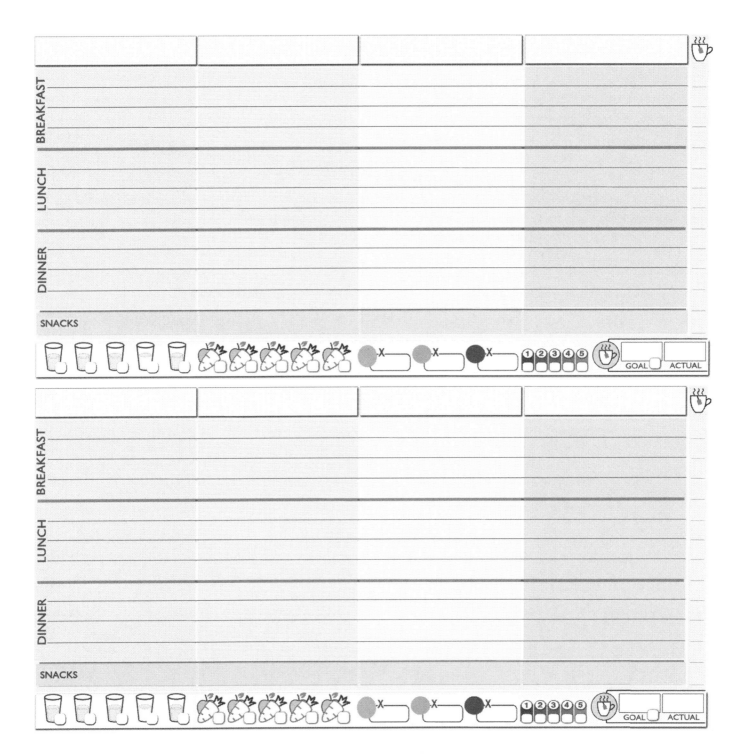

BREAKFAST

LUNCH

DINNER

SNACKS

GOAL   ACTUAL

BREAKFAST

LUNCH

DINNER

SNACKS

GOAL   ACTUAL

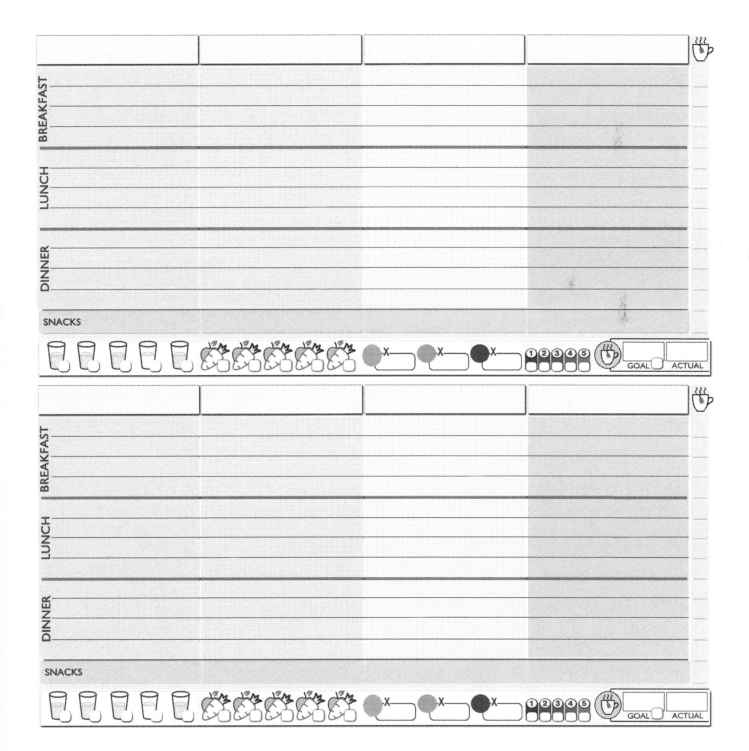

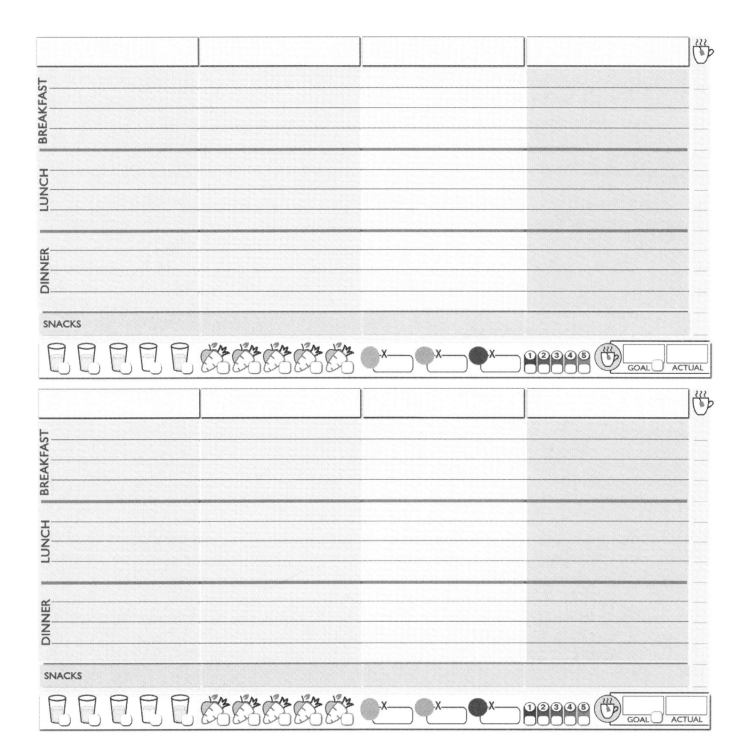

BREAKFAST

LUNCH

DINNER

SNACKS

GOAL ACTUAL

BREAKFAST

LUNCH

DINNER

SNACKS

GOAL ACTUAL

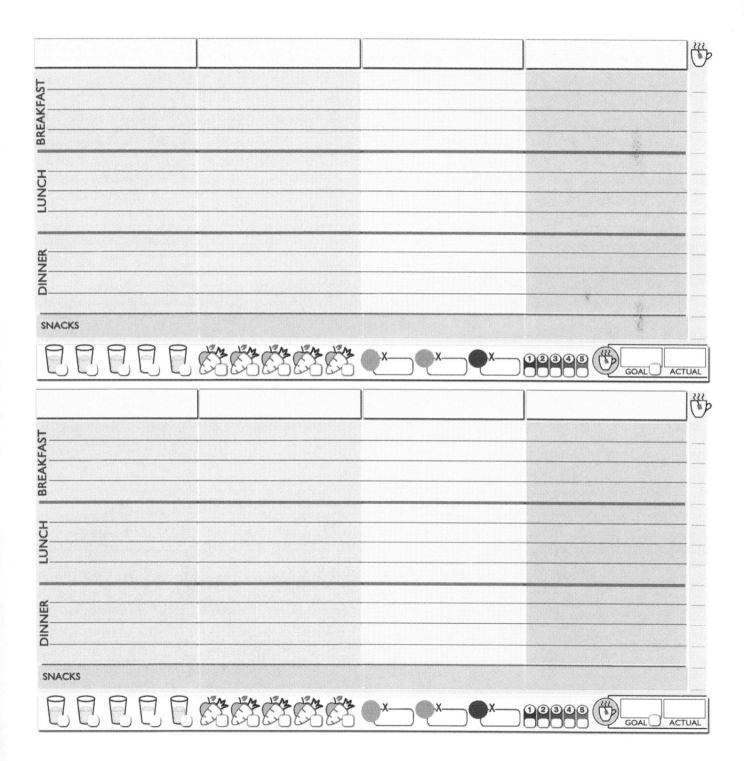

BREAKFAST

LUNCH

DINNER

SNACKS

GOAL · ACTUAL

BREAKFAST

LUNCH

DINNER

SNACKS

GOAL · ACTUAL

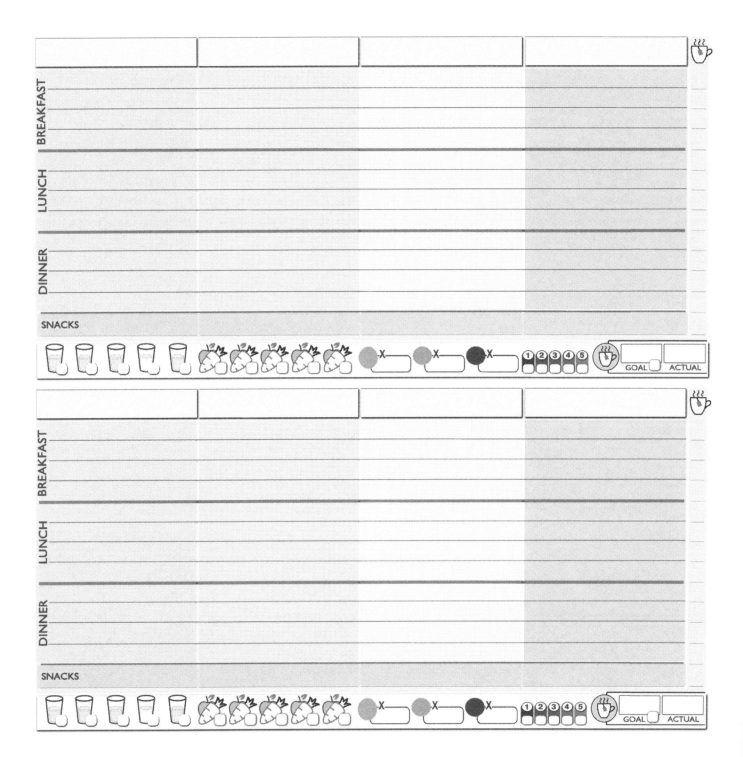

BREAKFAST

LUNCH

DINNER

SNACKS

GOAL   ACTUAL

BREAKFAST

LUNCH

DINNER

SNACKS

GOAL   ACTUAL

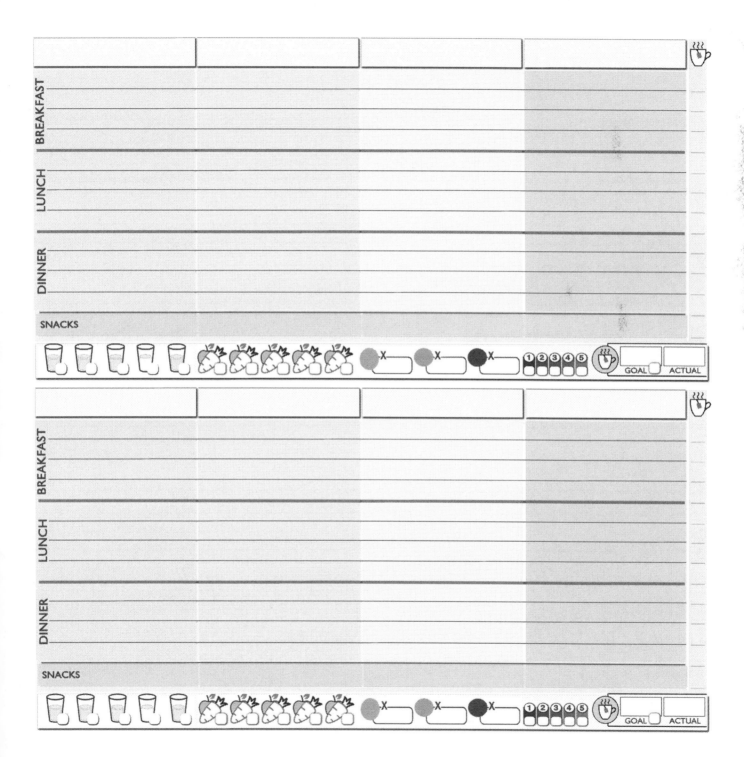

BREAKFAST

LUNCH

DINNER

SNACKS

GOAL   ACTUAL

BREAKFAST

LUNCH

DINNER

SNACKS

GOAL   ACTUAL

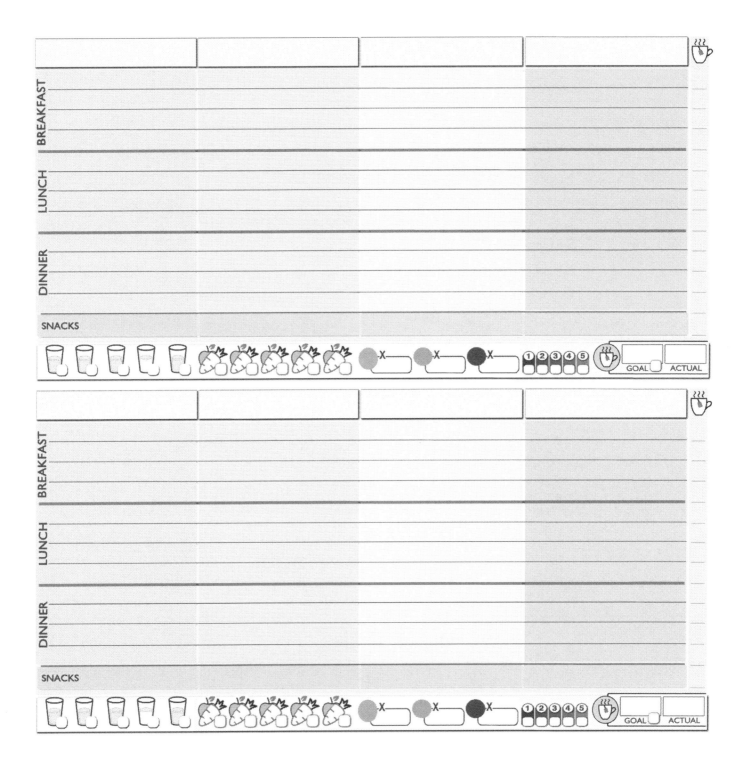

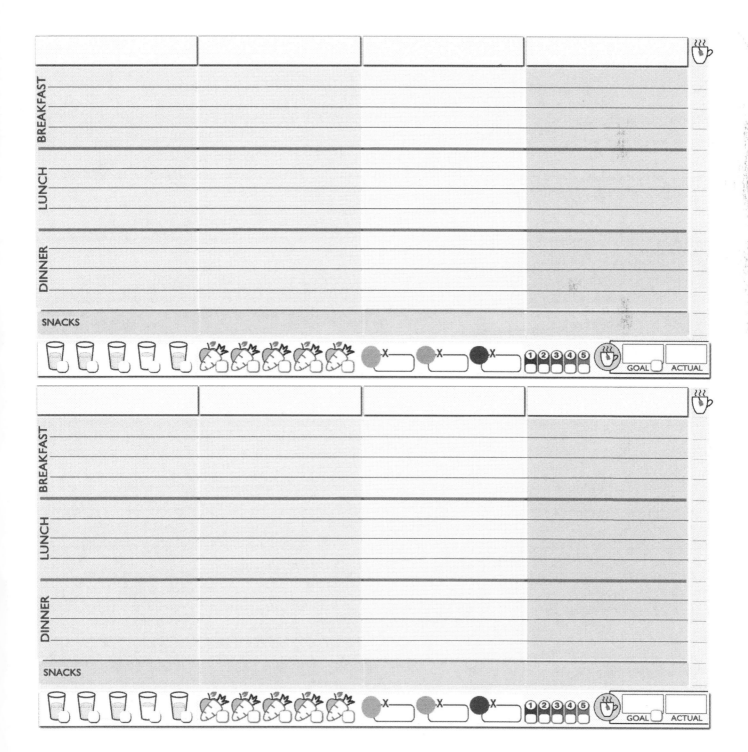

BREAKFAST

LUNCH

DINNER

SNACKS

GOAL ACTUAL

BREAKFAST

LUNCH

DINNER

SNACKS

GOAL ACTUAL

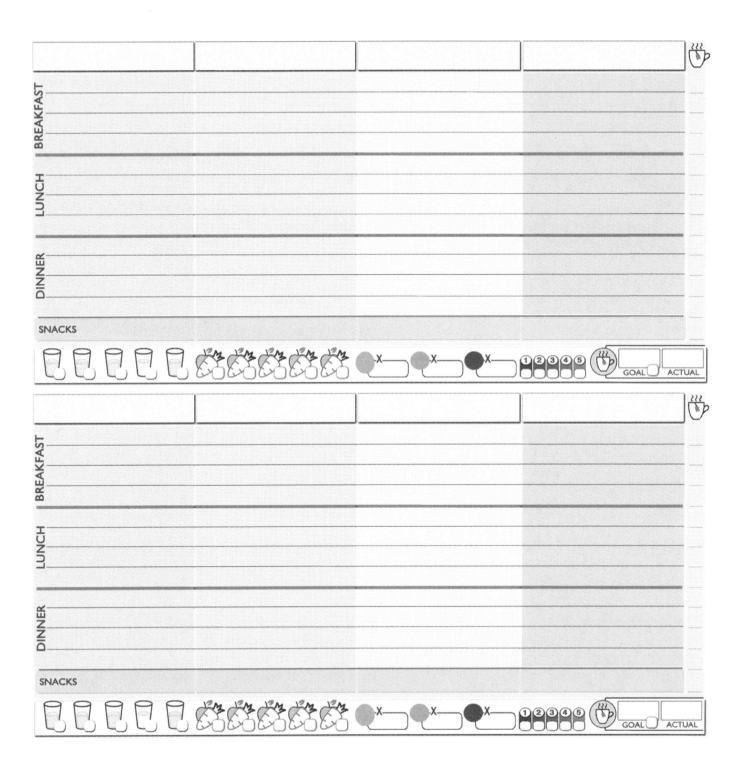

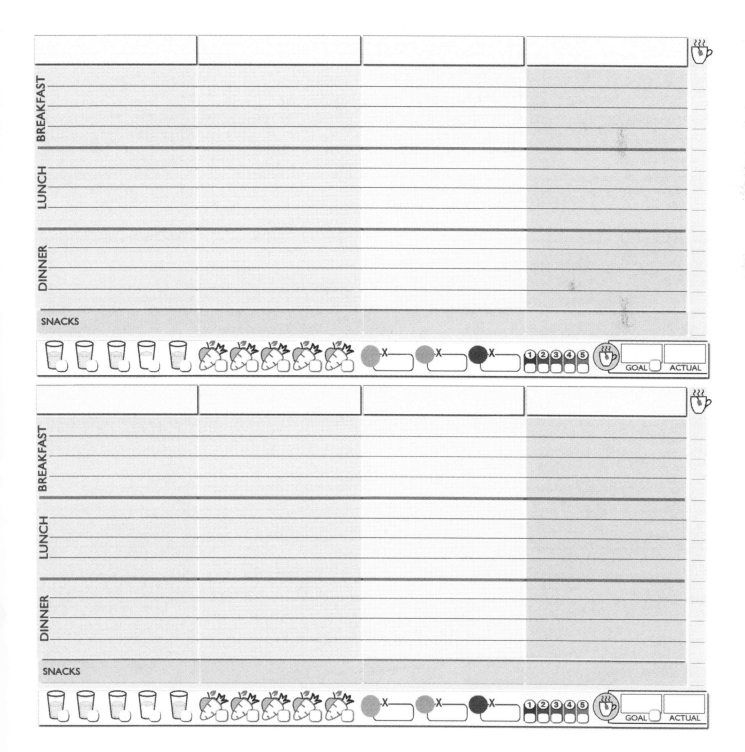

BREAKFAST

LUNCH

DINNER

SNACKS

GOAL ACTUAL

1 2 3 4 5

BREAKFAST

LUNCH

DINNER

SNACKS

GOAL ACTUAL

1 2 3 4 5

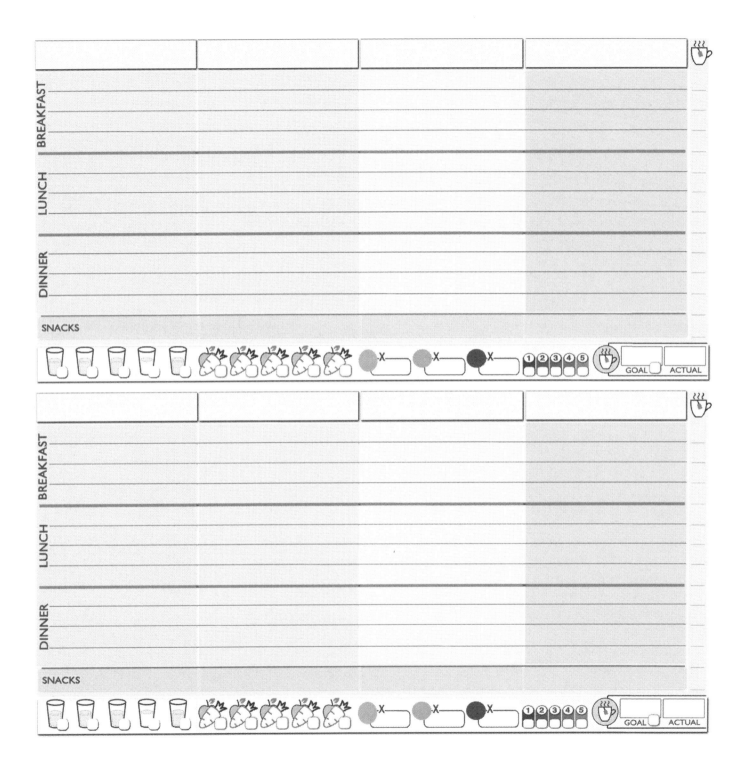

BREAKFAST

LUNCH

DINNER

SNACKS

1 2 3 4 5 GOAL ACTUAL

BREAKFAST

LUNCH

DINNER

SNACKS

1 2 3 4 5 GOAL ACTUAL

				☕
BREAKFAST				
LUNCH				
DINNER				
SNACKS				

🥛 🥛 🥛 🥛 🥛 🥕 🥕 🥕 🥕 🥕 ●—X ●—X ●—X ①②③④⑤ ☕ GOAL ☐ ACTUAL

				☕
BREAKFAST				
LUNCH				
DINNER				
SNACKS				

🥛 🥛 🥛 🥛 🥛 🥕 🥕 🥕 🥕 🥕 ●—X ●—X ●—X ①②③④⑤ ☕ GOAL ☐ ACTUAL

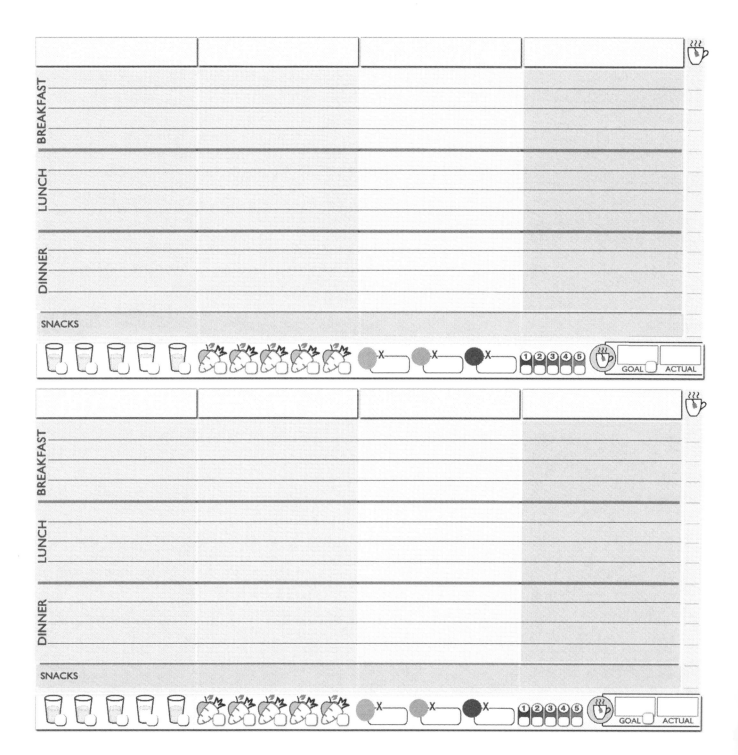

BREAKFAST

LUNCH

DINNER

SNACKS

GOAL   ACTUAL

BREAKFAST

LUNCH

DINNER

SNACKS

GOAL   ACTUAL

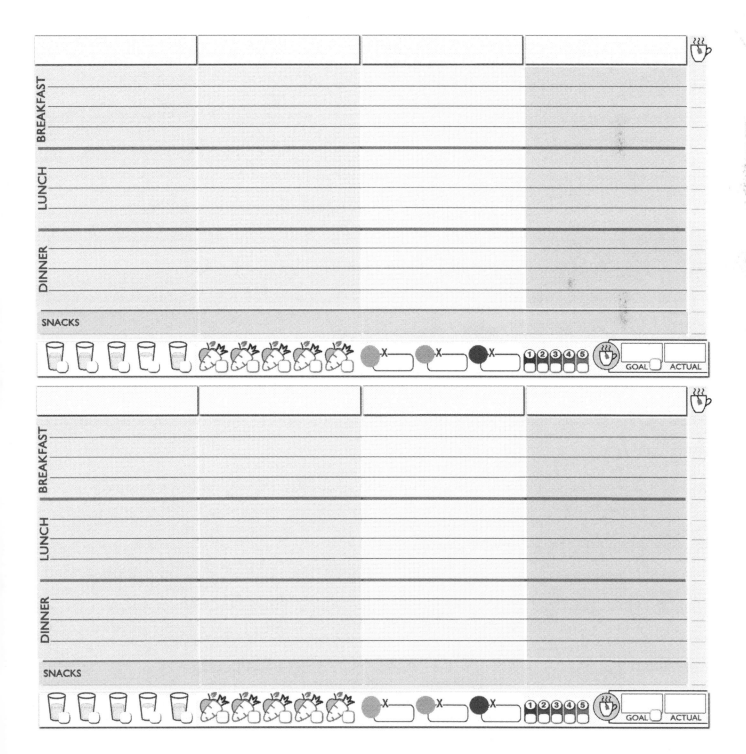

BREAKFAST

LUNCH

DINNER

SNACKS

GOAL   ACTUAL

BREAKFAST

LUNCH

DINNER

SNACKS

GOAL   ACTUAL

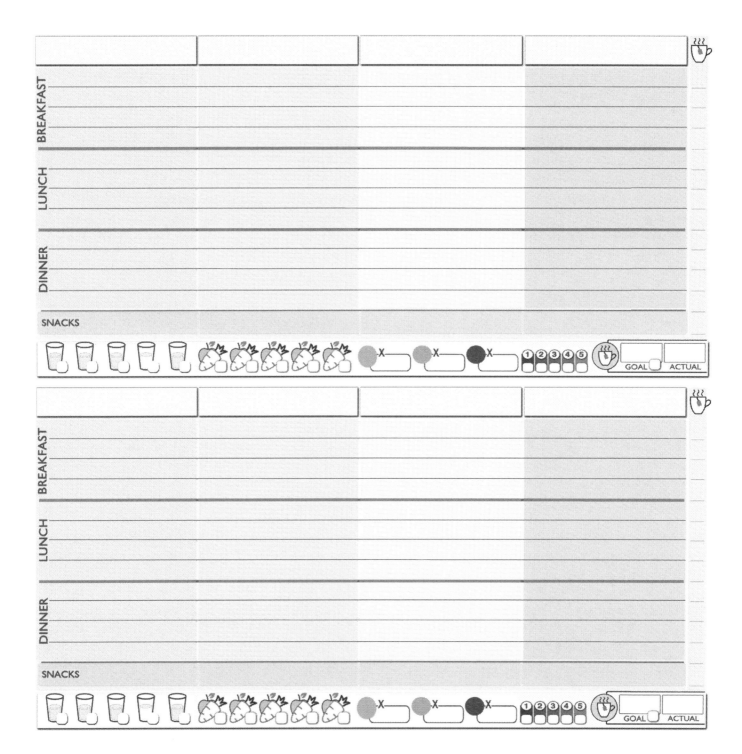

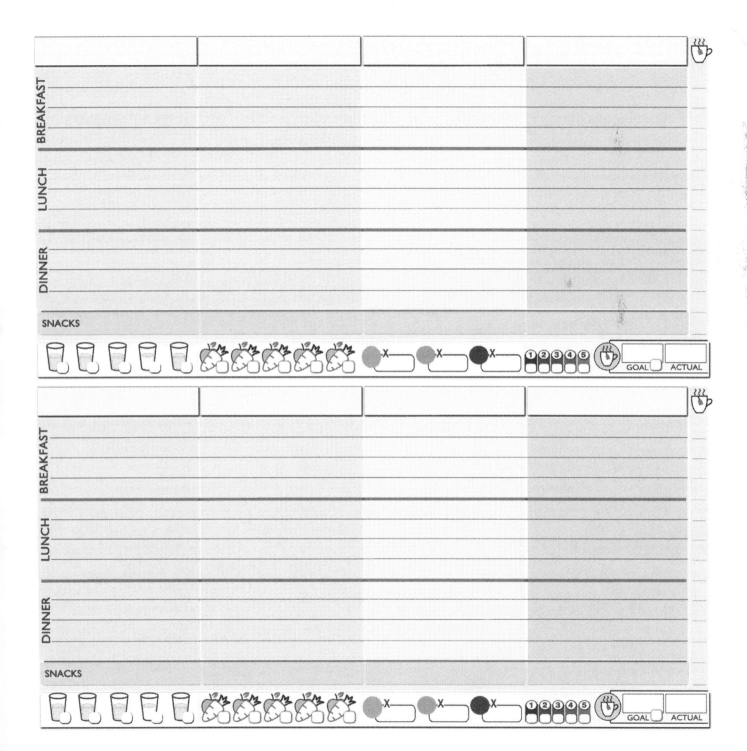

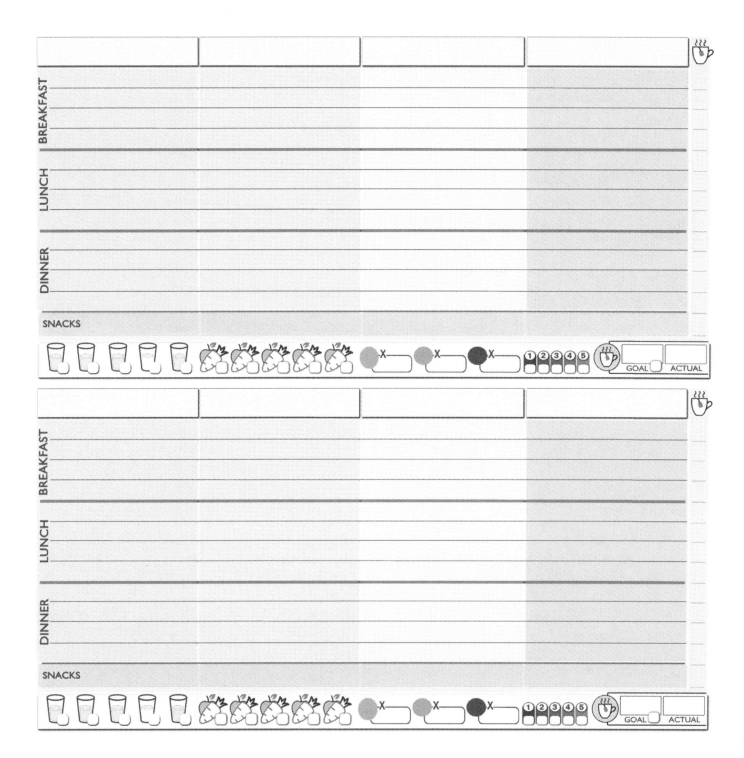

BREAKFAST

LUNCH

DINNER

SNACKS

GOAL   ACTUAL

BREAKFAST

LUNCH

DINNER

SNACKS

GOAL   ACTUAL

				☕
BREAKFAST				
LUNCH				
DINNER				
SNACKS				

🥛 🥛 🥛 🥛 🥛 🥕 🥕 🥕 🥕 🥕 ⬤X ⬤X ⬤X ①②③④⑤ ☕ GOAL ACTUAL

				☕
BREAKFAST				
LUNCH				
DINNER				
SNACKS				

🥛 🥛 🥛 🥛 🥛 🥕 🥕 🥕 🥕 🥕 ⬤X ⬤X ⬤X ①②③④⑤ ☕ GOAL ACTUAL

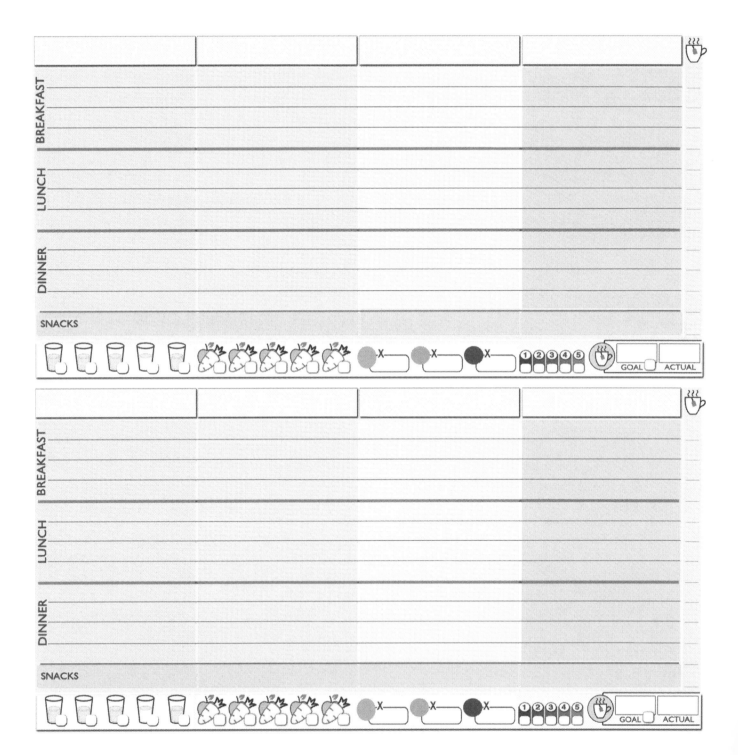

BREAKFAST

LUNCH

DINNER

SNACKS

GOAL ACTUAL

1 2 3 4 5

BREAKFAST

LUNCH

DINNER

SNACKS

GOAL ACTUAL

1 2 3 4 5

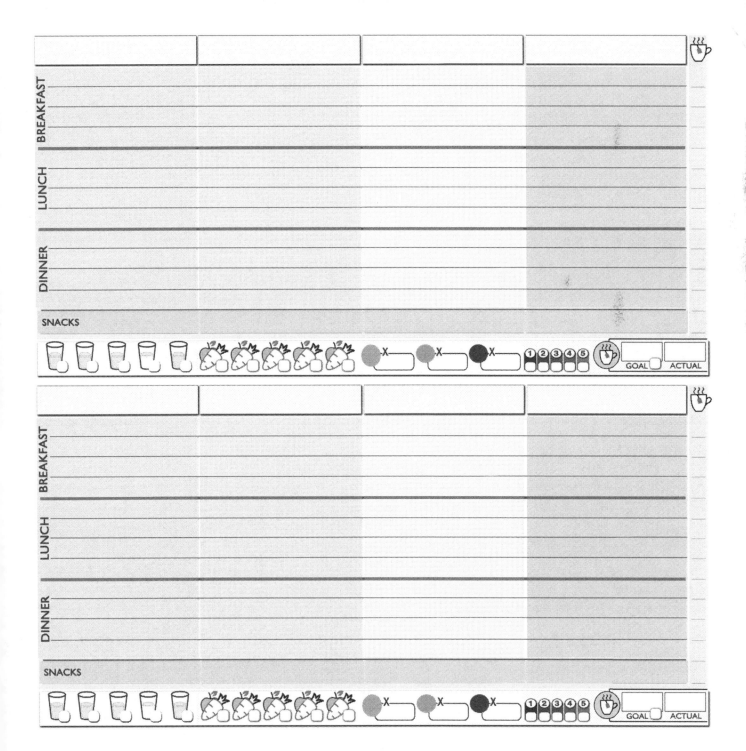

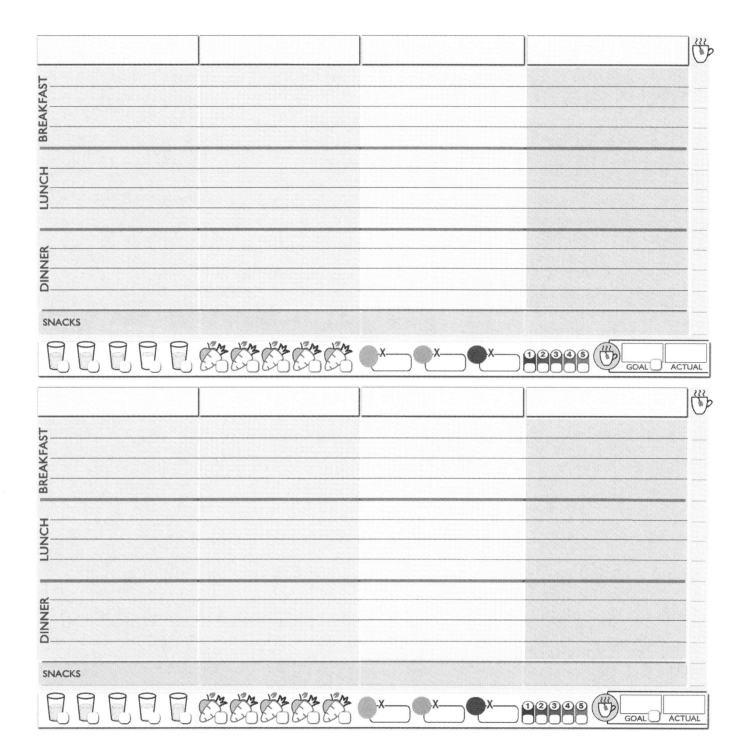

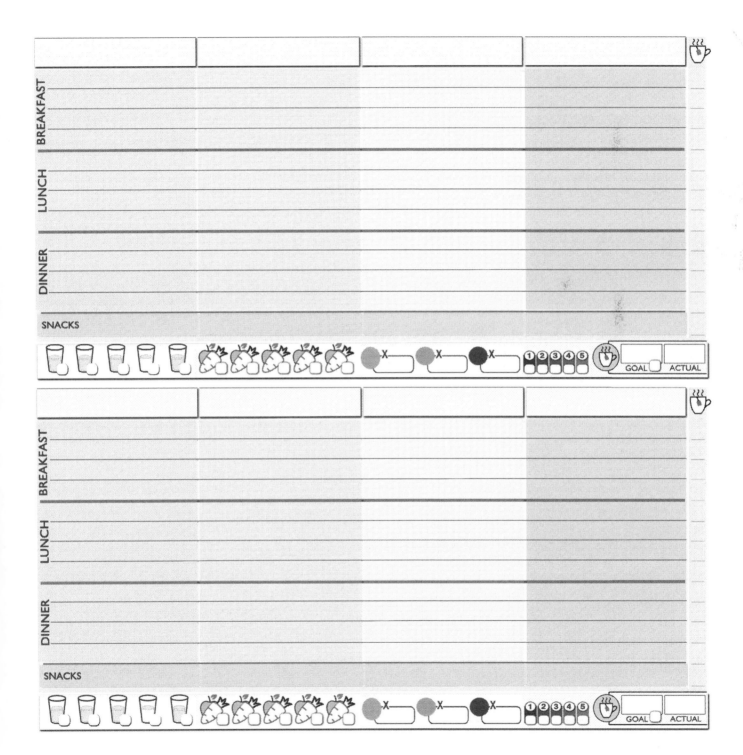

BREAKFAST

LUNCH

DINNER

SNACKS

GOAL   ACTUAL

BREAKFAST

LUNCH

DINNER

SNACKS

GOAL   ACTUAL

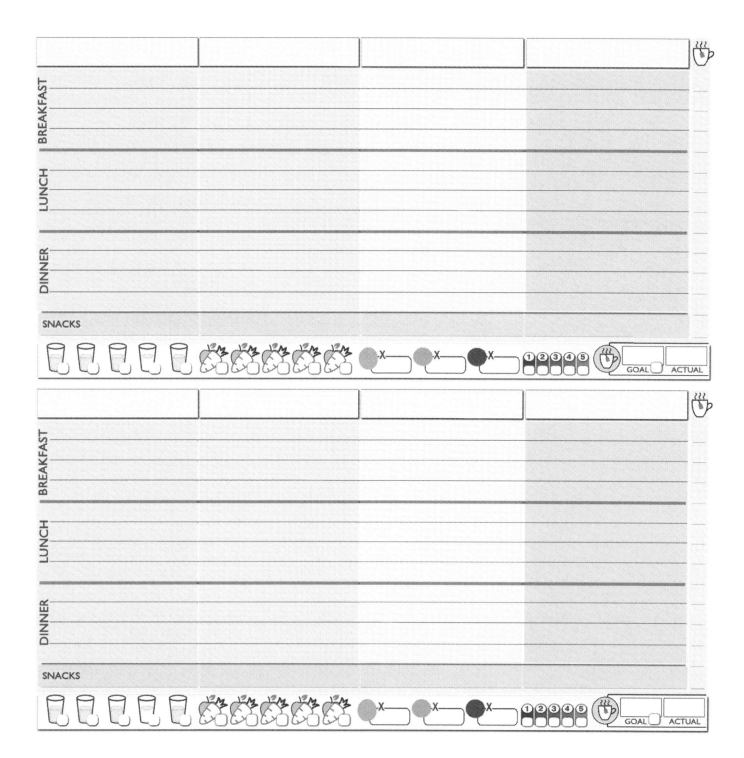

BREAKFAST

LUNCH

DINNER

SNACKS

GOAL   ACTUAL

BREAKFAST

LUNCH

DINNER

SNACKS

GOAL   ACTUAL

				☕

BREAKFAST

LUNCH

DINNER

SNACKS

GOAL   ACTUAL

				☕

BREAKFAST

LUNCH

DINNER

SNACKS

GOAL   ACTUAL

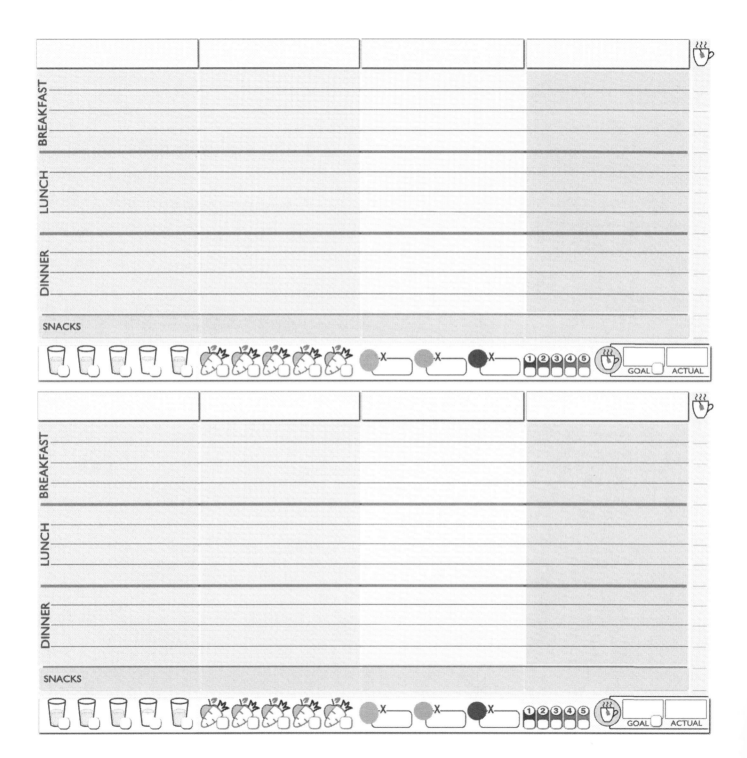

BREAKFAST

LUNCH

DINNER

SNACKS

GOAL   ACTUAL

BREAKFAST

LUNCH

DINNER

SNACKS

GOAL   ACTUAL

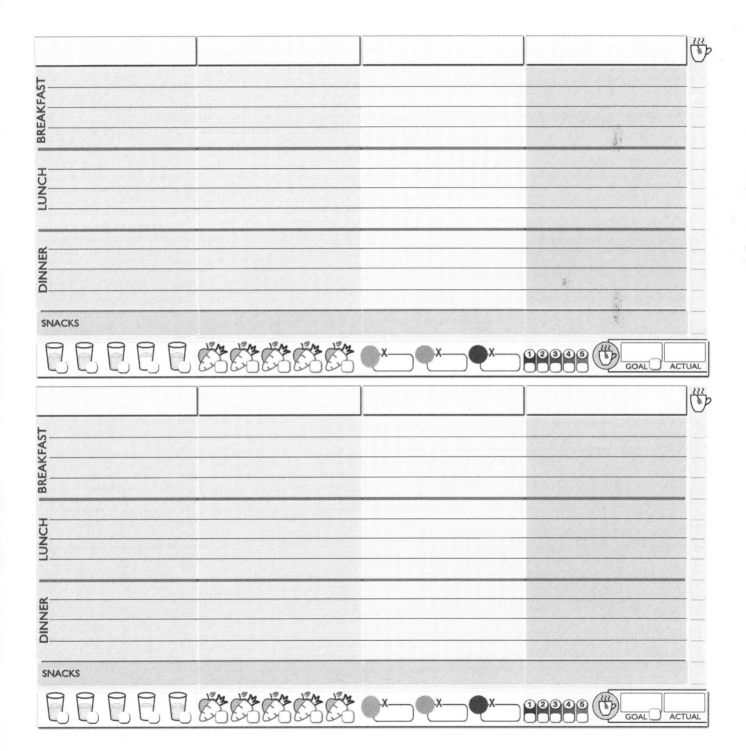

BREAKFAST

LUNCH

DINNER

SNACKS

GOAL   ACTUAL

BREAKFAST

LUNCH

DINNER

SNACKS

GOAL   ACTUAL

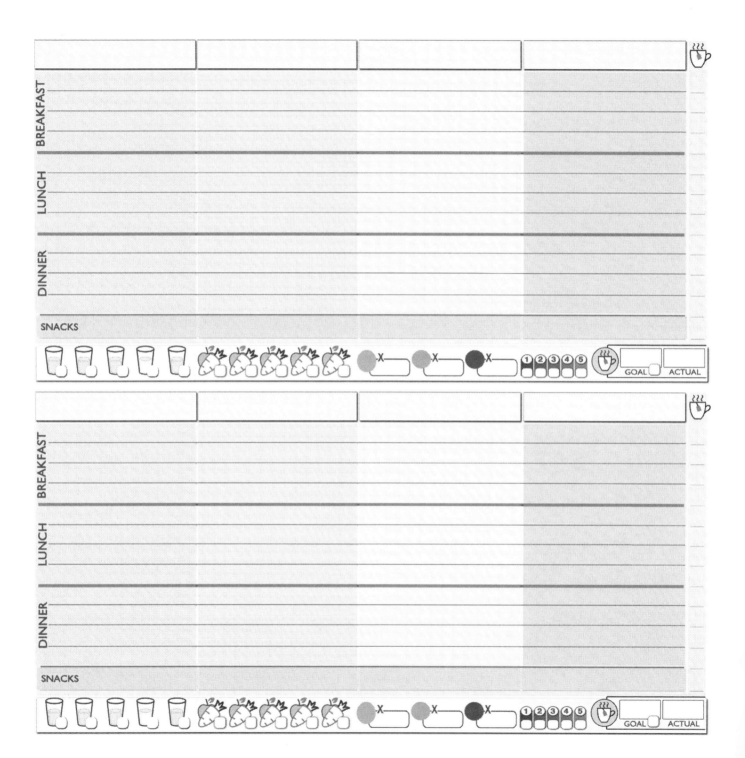

BREAKFAST

LUNCH

DINNER

SNACKS

GOAL   ACTUAL

BREAKFAST

LUNCH

DINNER

SNACKS

GOAL   ACTUAL

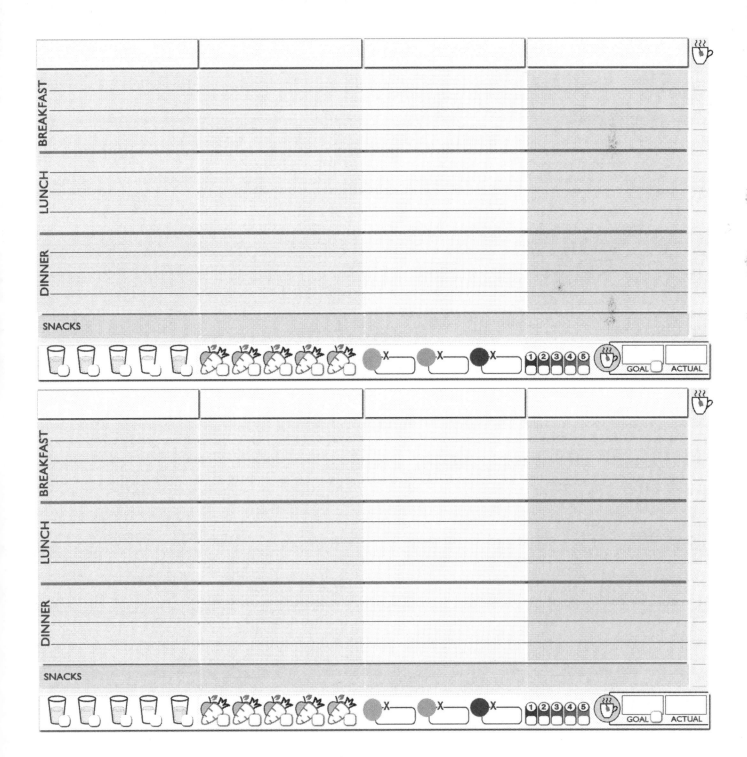

BREAKFAST

LUNCH

DINNER

SNACKS

GOAL   ACTUAL

BREAKFAST

LUNCH

DINNER

SNACKS

GOAL   ACTUAL

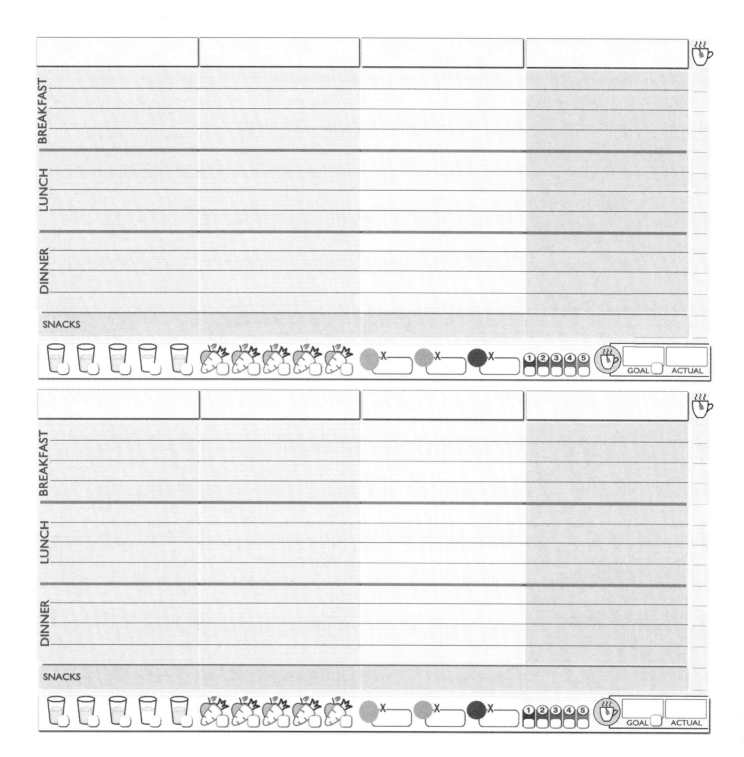

WHY DO WE NEED TO EXERCISE

Exercising makes us fit and healthy. It's what we do, to simulate what our ancestors did a long time ago. Some people don't have to exercise at all because their day to day activities are just so energy demanding, they can eat as much and as often as they like and look pretty fit, trim and healthy. These individuals have found their body balance. The energy (Calories) they consume is equal to the energy (Calories) they burn.

These individuals are usually heavy labourers and are constantly using their muscles. For the rest of us to get to the same level of energy output, we have to play sports or hit the gym and exercise!

Sometimes it's forgotten what exercising is all about! It is often thought of as a sport people do simply for fun and to look good. But if you really think about it, it is an essential way of life. If your day to day living is not burning off the energy (Calories) you consume, then it's something you have to do to keep your body balanced. And if you don't, well you know what happens!

There are a number of reasons why we don't all have gym memberships; "It's not my thing", "I can't afford it", "I'm not fit enough", "I don't have time", "I don't want to look silly", "I can't perform those exercises". The list is long!

And working out at home can sometimes offer up even more reasons not to be doing it. Sometimes the intention is there and the motivation simply isn't. That's why many of us have dusty exercise bikes in the corner of the room, doubling up as a clothes horse! You need motivation and a solid reason to exercise five days per week and because you don't have a personal trainer knocking on your door at 7.30am, it's all up to you! Now you have the reason, you simply need the motivation.

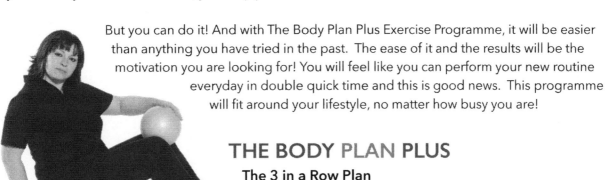

But you can do it! And with The Body Plan Plus Exercise Programme, it will be easier than anything you have tried in the past. The ease of it and the results will be the motivation you are looking for! You will feel like you can perform your new routine everyday in double quick time and this is good news. This programme will fit around your lifestyle, no matter how busy you are!

THE BODY PLAN PLUS
The 3 in a Row Plan

Diets and Exercising do not fail, they work! What fails us is our starting point. If you do something your body isn't used to, it will simply tire. You get all the signals rushing to your brain telling us, "This is to much", "I don't like it", and "Don't do it again".

You get these signals, (Feelings) because you try to do something your body isn't ready for yet. To prepare your body for anything, you have to do it at a pace that allows it to adapt! You have to do something that is easy, and not too taxing for you, emotionally as well as physically.

A little scenario for you to prove my point! If you had a magic red button and to lose a pound of body fat each week, all you had to do is push it repeatedly for 20 minutes last thing at night Would you push it? Of course you would, and you would not miss a single day until your goal weight was reached! And why would you never miss a day? Because it's so easy and effortless!

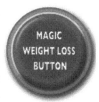

So! We have now proven, if it's easy, you will do it again and again until your goals are reached. We have also learnt you are prepared to dedicate 20 minutes of your time for the task.

But how can we make exercising easy? "It's hard isn't it? I've seen people jumping around like they are on fire" and that looks difficult! These individuals are not on fire, they have simply reached a level where, what they are doing is still quite easy to them, and they feel good about it. But they too had a starting point!

It's all about the starting point and what your body is capable of doing! You need to do something slowly and at a pace your body will thank you for. And if you do, you will get the right signals rushing to your brain - "This is easy", "This is fun", "I feel good", "I want to do it again" "I feel motivated"!

The exercise formula we have created is called "**The 3 in a Row Plan**" It's the best exercise formula ever and it's for everyone! Regardless of your current weight, fitness level, stamina or flexibility this plan will work for you.

The "**3 in a Row Pan**" allows your body time to adapt to the small changes, and pushing your body to the next level when its ready to.... thus making it as easy as pushing a magic button.

For more information and to watch our short video about this amazing exercise plan, please visit:
www.thebodyplanplus.com

Personally I have been on my own weight loss journey... And from the journey, came knowledge that created this business. My aim is to help others reach their goals and provide them with the tools needed to help complete their journeys.

This Diary has been created and designed so it is compatible with any dieting or food plan. Following a main stream diet plan is not the way I lost my weight, but I cant twist everyones arm to follow my way.

But I can show you my way, and you can make up your own mind!

Welcome to The Body Plan Plus TM

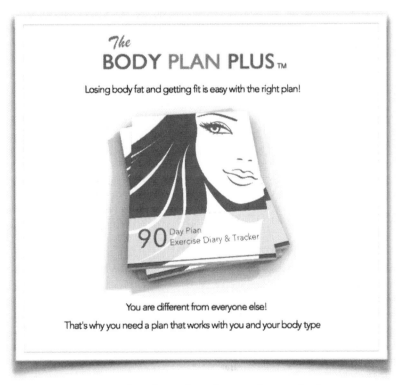

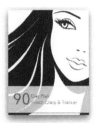
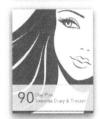
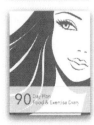

Which Plan is For You?

You don't need to pay a monthly club fee to lose weight.

You simply need one of three clever books - Plain and Simple!

Do you need a Food Plan, an Exercise Plan or a little of Both?

Visit our website, watch the videos and you decide...!

www.thebodyplanplus.club

35539915R00040

Printed in Poland
by Amazon Fulfillment
Poland Sp. z o.o., Wrocław